COMPLETE GUIDE TO UNDERSTANDING VASECTOMY

Everything You Need To Know About Male Sterilization, Procedure, Recovery, Risks, Benefits, Post-Op Care For Informed Decision-Making And Long-Term Health.

KLEIN HOYLE

© [KLEIN HOYLE] [2024]

All rights reserved.

No part of this book may be reproduced, distributed, or transmitted in any form or by any means, including photocopying, recording, or other electronic or mechanical methods, without the publisher's prior written permission, with the exception of brief quotations in critical reviews and certain other noncommercial uses permitted by copyright law.

Disclaimer

The content in this book is based on the author's expertise and comprehension of the topic. The author has no affiliation or link with any corporation, business, or person. This book is meant to give general information and educational material only, and it should not be interpreted as professional medical advice. Always seek the advice of a skilled healthcare expert if you have any queries about medical issues or treatments. The author and publisher expressly disclaim any responsibility resulting directly or indirectly from the use or use of the information included in this book.

Table of Contents

CHAPTER 1 13
Introduction To Vasectomy 13
What Is A Vasectomy? 13
History And Evolution Of Vasectomy 13
Reasons To Consider Vasectomy....................14
Myths And Misconceptions Regarding Vasectomy
....15

CHAPTER 2 17
Understanding Male Reproductive Anatomy.....17
An Overview Of The Male Reproductive System 17
Detailed Explanation Of The Vas Deferens.......18
The Role Of Sperm In Reproduction 19
How Does Vasectomy Affect Sperm Flow 20

CHAPTER 3 23
Preparing For Vasectomy 23
Consult With A Healthcare Provider 23
Preoperative Instructions And Preparations 24
   1. Avoiding specific medications:................25
   2. Shaving the genital region:......................25
   3. Arrange transportation: 25

    4. Fasting before the procedure: 25
    Mental And Emotional Readiness 26
    Discussing Vasectomy With Your Partner 27
CHAPTER 4 29
    Types Of Vasectomy Procedures 29
    Traditional Vasectomy Technique 29
    No-Scalpel Vasectomy 30
    Differences And Similarities Between Techniques
    31
    Advantages And Disadvantages Of Each
    Procedure 32
CHAPTER 5 35
    Vasectomy Procedure 35
    Step-By-Step Guide To Vasectomy Surgery 35
        1. Preparation: 35
        2. Anesthetic: 35
        3. Sterilization: 36
        4. Vasectomy: 36
        5. Closure: 36
        6. Recovery: 36
        7. Follow-Up: 37

Anesthesia Options And Pain Management 37
    1. Local Anesthesia: 38
    2. Conscious Sedation: 38
    3. General Anesthesia: 38

Possible Dangers And Issues 39
    1. Bleeding: 39
    3. Chronic Pain: 40
    4. Sperm Granuloma: 40
    5. Sperm Regrowth: 41

Post-Procedure Care Instructions 41
    1. Rest and Recovery: 41
    2. Ice Packs: 42
    3. Pain Relief: 42
    6. Follow-up visit: 43

CHAPTER 6 45
Recovery And Aftercare 45
Immediate Postoperative Care 45
Overcoming Pain And Uncomfort 46
Resuming Normal Activity 47
Long-Term Concerns For Sexual Health 48

CHAPTER 7 51

Possible Dangers And Issues 51
Common Risks Associated With Vasectomy 51
Rare Complications And How To Treat Them ... 52
Signs Of Postoperative Complications 53
When To Seek Medical Attention? 54

CHAPTER 8 57

Vasectomy Reversal 57
Overview Of The Vasectomy Reversal Procedure
.... 57
Success Rates And Factors Impacting Outcomes 58
Alternatives For Vasectomy Reversal 59
Emotional And Psychological Implications Of
Reversal 60

CHAPTER 9 63

Vasectomy Myths Busted 63
Addressing Common Misconceptions About
Vasectomy 63

Myth 1: A vasectomy causes erectile dysfunction
.... 63
Myth 2: Vasectomy reduces sexual pleasure 64
Myth 3: Vasectomy is irreversible 64

Myth 4: Vasectomy increases the risk of prostate cancer 65
Distinguishing Fact From Fiction 65
Clarifying Doubts And Concerns 66
Promoting Informed Decision-Making 66
CHAPTER 10 67
Life Following Vasectomy 67
Adjusting To Life After Vasectomy 67
Effect On Sexual Health And Intimacy 69
Family Planning Considerations 70
Conclusion 73
THE END 76

ABOUT THIS BOOK

The "Complete Guide to Understanding Vasectomy" is an invaluable resource for anybody contemplating or receiving a vasectomy, covering a wide range of key topics in a thorough but understandable way.

The opening chapters provide readers with insight into the core of vasectomy, delving into its historical background and development while refuting common myths and misunderstandings about the treatment. Understanding the importance of vasectomy is critical, and this section provides a good basis for making educated decisions.

This book then delves into the complexities of male reproductive anatomy, explaining the importance of each component in fertility and how vasectomy disrupts sperm flow. This awareness is critical for persons considering vasectomy because it provides them with knowledge about the physiological ramifications of the surgery.

Preparation is essential, and This book thoroughly discusses pre-operative issues such as talks with healthcare specialists, mental preparedness, and conversations with partners. Such preparation promotes a comprehensive approach to vasectomy, ensuring that people are emotionally and practically prepared for the path ahead.

A thorough examination of vasectomy procedures follows, comparing conventional methods to current options such as the no-scalpel approach. By outlining the benefits and downsides of each approach, readers can make educated decisions based on their tastes and requirements.

The procedural element of vasectomy is thoroughly explored, offering a step-by-step summary of the procedure, anesthetic alternatives, and post-operative care instructions. Potential dangers and problems are also openly explored, providing readers with the information they need to confidently navigate the recovery process.

In terms of recovery, This book includes a section on post-operative care, which provides practical advice for dealing with pain and returning to regular activities. Long-term sexual health issues are also addressed, ensuring that patients are prepared to negotiate the post-vasectomy environment successfully.

Furthermore, This book dives into possible hazards and problems, preparing readers to detect warning signals and seek immediate medical assistance if required. Furthermore, it delves into the complex issue of vasectomy reversal, offering information on success rates, alternatives, and the emotional journey connected with reversal surgeries.

Dispelling myths and misunderstandings is critical, and This book includes a section dispelling common falsehoods about vasectomy. Separating reality from fantasy empowers readers to make truth-based judgments, supporting educated decision-making and removing unfounded anxieties.

Finally, This book provides insights into life following a vasectomy, including changes, effects on sexual health and intimacy, and family planning options. By providing a comprehensive overview of the post-vasectomy world, it gives readers the skills they need to confidently navigate this new chapter of their lives.

CHAPTER 1

Introduction To Vasectomy

What Is A Vasectomy?

Vasectomy, often known as male sterilization, is a surgical technique used to offer permanent contraception for males. During the surgery, the vas deferens, which transports sperm from the testicles to the urethra, are severed, sealed, or obstructed. This inhibits sperm from reaching the semen ejaculated from the penis, thereby rendering the guy infertile.

History And Evolution Of Vasectomy

Vasectomy has a centuries-long history, with early types of male sterilization treatments discovered in ancient civilizations such as China and India. However, contemporary vasectomy procedures emerged in the early twentieth century. In 1899, a physician called Harry Sharp conducted the first documented vasectomy in the United States. Since then, advances in surgical procedures and technology have made vasectomy a safe and popular form of contraception.

Reasons To Consider Vasectomy

There are a variety of reasons why individuals or couples may choose vasectomy as a contraception method. One of the main reasons is its efficacy. Vasectomy is one of the most effective ways of contraception, with a success rate of more than 99%. It also provides a permanent answer to contraception, removing the need for continuous contraceptive methods like condoms or chemical birth control. Some people may choose vasectomy for personal or medical reasons, such as avoiding the hazards of female sterilization or stopping the spread of hereditary diseases.

Myths And Misconceptions Regarding Vasectomy

Despite its efficiency and safety, vasectomy is often associated with myths and misunderstandings, which might discourage people from considering it as an option. One prevalent misconception is that vasectomy impairs sexual performance or desire. In truth, vasectomy does not affect a man's ability to have an erection or enjoy sexual intercourse. Another myth is that a vasectomy is a painful or complex surgery. While pain during and after the treatment is natural, advances in surgical procedures have made vasectomy very rapid and simple, with little downtime.

Understanding these characteristics of vasectomy is critical to making an educated choice about whether it is the best contraception option for you. Individuals may approach vasectomy with confidence and clarity if myths and misunderstandings are dispelled, as well as the history and reasons for contemplating it.

CHAPTER 2

Understanding Male Reproductive Anatomy

An Overview Of The Male Reproductive System

The male reproductive system is a biological wonder, engineered to generate, nourish, and transport sperm—the microscopic fertilization agents that launch the process of creating new life. This system is built around a few main components, each of which plays an important function in the overall process.

First and foremost are the testes, sometimes known as the "gonads" of the male reproductive system. These produce both sperm and testosterone, the key male sex hormone. The testes are encased inside the scrotum and dangle outside the body to maintain a lower temperature that is ideal for sperm production.

The epididymis and vas deferens are two structures that connect to the testes. The epididymis stores and matures sperm, enabling them to become motile and fertile. The vas deferens, which is sometimes compared to a muscle highway, then transfer sperm from the epididymis to the ejaculatory ducts during ejaculation.

These structures are accompanied by auxiliary glands, such as seminal vesicles and the prostate gland. These glands create seminal fluid, a nutrient-dense medium that feeds and protects sperm during ejaculation. Finally, the urethra serves as the channel via which urine and sperm escape the body.

Detailed Explanation Of The Vas Deferens

The vas deferens, also known as the ductus deferens, is a small muscular tube used to transfer sperm. The vas deferens, which extends from the epididymis to the ejaculatory ducts, are essential for ejaculation.

Its structure is made up of smooth muscle fibers, which enable it to contract and drive sperm forward during ejaculation. This muscularity also helps to regulate sperm flow, resulting in a constant stream during ejaculation.

In addition to its transit role, the vas deferens has an epithelial cell lining that secretes chemicals to feed and protect the sperm as it travels to its destination. This lining also helps to maintain proper pH levels, which are important for sperm survival.

The Role Of Sperm In Reproduction

Sperm, the tiny cells generated by the male reproductive system, are the primary participants in sexual reproduction. Each sperm cell includes the genetic material required for fertilization, including DNA packed inside the head region.

Sperm's voyage starts in the seminiferous tubules of the testes, where it goes through a process known as spermatogenesis. Spermatogonia, which are diploid cells, divide and develop into mature sperm cells by mitotic and meiotic divisions.

Once formed, sperm move through the epididymis, maturing and gaining motility—a necessary condition for their function in fertilization. During ejaculation, sperm travel via the vas deferens and combine with seminal fluid from the accessory glands to generate semen.

When sperm enter the female reproductive canal by ejaculation, they race towards the egg to fertilize it. This voyage is fraught with challenges, such as acidic conditions and physical barriers, yet the sperm's resilience permits some to arrive and fertilize.

How Does Vasectomy Affect Sperm Flow

Vasectomy, a surgical treatment used for male sterilization, inhibits the passage of sperm via the vas deferens, thereby stopping their release during ejaculation. This is accomplished by cutting, sealing, or obstructing the vas deferens, creating a physical barrier that keeps sperm from mingling with semen.

Fertilization cannot occur in the absence of sperm in the ejaculate, making the person essentially infertile. However, it is important to highlight that vasectomy has no effect on testicular sperm generation or seminal fluid secretion by the accessory glands. As a result, sexual function and ejaculation remain unaltered after the treatment.

Despite its efficacy, vasectomy is considered a permanent method of contraception and should be done with caution. While reversal techniques are available, they are not always effective, thus vasectomy represents a long-term commitment to contraception.

CHAPTER 3

Preparing For Vasectomy

Consult With A Healthcare Provider

Before having a vasectomy, it is essential to speak with a healthcare professional. This first step is critical for comprehending the procedure, and its effects, and determining whether it's the best option for you. During this appointment, the healthcare practitioner will review your medical history, address any concerns or questions you may have, and offer full information regarding the vasectomy procedure.

The healthcare practitioner will also do a physical examination to determine your general health and appropriateness for the treatment. This evaluation may involve monitoring your blood pressure, examining any medicines you are presently taking, and addressing any allergies or pre-existing diseases that may interfere with the treatment or recovery.

Furthermore, the consultation provides a chance to discuss your reproductive objectives and if a vasectomy is appropriate for your family planning needs. To obtain the best advice and assistance, you must be open and honest throughout this conversation.

Preoperative Instructions And Preparations

Once you have chosen to have a vasectomy, your healthcare professional will provide you with pre-operative instructions to follow. These recommendations are intended to assist in ensuring the procedure's success while reducing the chance of problems.

Common pre-operative instructions might include:

1. Avoiding specific medications: Your doctor may urge you to avoid taking blood thinners such as aspirin or ibuprofen in the days leading up to the operation to lessen the risk of severe bleeding during and after the vasectomy.

2. Shaving the genital region: Before the operation, you may be told to shave the genital area to increase visibility and cleanliness during the surgery.

3. Arrange transportation: Because vasectomy is usually done under local anesthetic, you may be able to drive yourself to and from the appointment. However, if you have any pain or dizziness as a result of the surgery, you should make arrangements for transportation back home.

4. Fasting before the procedure: Your healthcare professional may advise you to fast for a certain length of time before the vasectomy, particularly if general anesthesia will be utilized.

Follow these pre-operative guidelines carefully to ensure a smooth and successful vasectomy treatment.

Mental And Emotional Readiness

A vasectomy is an emotional as well as a physical procedure. It's critical to psychologically prepare oneself for the surgery and its possible consequences.

Many men feel a variety of emotions before a vasectomy, including fear, uncertainty, and even melancholy. These are perfectly natural sentiments that should be recognized and dealt with freely.

One method to psychologically prepare for a vasectomy is to extensively research the process. Understanding how the vasectomy works, what to anticipate during and after the surgery, and the possible long-term consequences might help to reduce fear and uncertainty.

Furthermore, addressing your emotions with your healthcare professional, trustworthy friends, or family members may give vital support and comfort at this time.

Discussing Vasectomy With Your Partner

If you're in a committed relationship, you should openly discuss your desire to get a vasectomy with your spouse. This discussion should include you revealing your reasons for contemplating the surgery, answering any worries or questions your partner may have, and talking about how the choice may affect your relationship and future family planning.

Open communication is essential for making both partners feel heard, supported, and participated in the decision-making process. Your spouse may have different views and sentiments regarding vasectomy, so approach the subject with respect and compassion.

Furthermore, including your spouse in the decision-making process may enhance your bond and promote a feeling of shared responsibility for family planning.

By discussing vasectomy openly and honestly with your spouse, you can guarantee that you are both on the same page and ready to proceed with the operation together.

CHAPTER 4

Types Of Vasectomy Procedures

Traditional Vasectomy Technique

The conventional vasectomy procedure, commonly known as the incision method, is among the earliest techniques of male sterilization. In this surgery, the doctor makes one or two tiny incisions in the scrotum to get access to the vas deferens, which transports sperm from the testicles to the urethra. To prevent sperm from passing through the vas deferens, they are cut, tied up, or sealed.

This surgery is usually conducted under local anesthetic, which means the patient is awake but not in pain in the region being operated on. The incisions are minor and often need stitches to seal. Recovery times vary from person to person, but they often last a few days to a week.

While the classic vasectomy procedure has been routinely used for many years and is regarded as successful, it does have certain drawbacks. The incisions produced during the surgery may occasionally result in consequences including infection, bleeding, or bruising. Furthermore, since the incisions are done directly in the scrotum, there is a danger of injuring adjacent tissues or structures.

No-Scalpel Vasectomy

The no-scalpel vasectomy, or NSV, is a more recent procedure that was created to solve some of the drawbacks of the old approach. The doctor punctures the scrotum skin with a specific device rather than making incisions with a knife. The hole is then expanded to provide access to the vas deferens.

One of the primary benefits of the no-scalpel vasectomy is that it is less invasive than the conventional procedure. No incisions are created, thus there is minimal bleeding, bruising, and infection risk.

Punctures also heal faster than incisions, allowing the patient to recuperate more quickly.

The no-scalpel vasectomy is not only less invasive, but it also takes less time to do. The complete operation normally takes 20-30 minutes, as opposed to 30-45 minutes with the old approach. This may be more convenient for both the patient and the physician.

Differences And Similarities Between Techniques

While both classic vasectomy and no-scalpel vasectomy are effective techniques of male sterilization, they vary in numerous significant respects. The most evident difference is how the process is executed; one requires making tiny incisions in the scrotum, while the other employs a puncture approach.

The no-scalpel vasectomy has the benefit of being less intrusive and requiring a shorter recovery period.

However, other research has revealed that the two procedures may not vary much in terms of long-term results or complication rates.

It's also worth mentioning that both treatments are often regarded as very successful in avoiding pregnancy. Following any kind of vasectomy, men should continue to take contraception until a follow-up test reveals that no sperm is present in their sperm.

Advantages And Disadvantages Of Each Procedure

The classic vasectomy approach has the benefit of being a long-standing method that has been used effectively for many years. It is effective in preventing pregnancy and quite straightforward to carry out. However, it has significant disadvantages, including the possibility of problems such as infection or bleeding, as well as a lengthier recovery period.

On the other side, the no-scalpel vasectomy has significant benefits over the conventional approach. It is less intrusive, which may result in less pain and a quicker recovery for the patient. It is also faster to do, which benefits both the patient and the doctor. However, it may not be appropriate for all guys, especially those with certain anatomical difficulties.

Finally, the particular patient's wishes and circumstances will determine whether to do a regular vasectomy or a no-scalpel vasectomy. Men wanting a vasectomy should consult with a knowledgeable healthcare expert to establish which surgery is best for them.

CHAPTER 5

Vasectomy Procedure

Step-By-Step Guide To Vasectomy Surgery

When it comes to vasectomy surgery, knowing the step-by-step procedure will help relieve any concerns. Here is a summary of what you may expect:

1. Preparation: Before the surgery starts, your doctor will go over your medical history and any drugs you are presently taking. To protect your safety before surgery, you must give any relevant information, such as allergies or pre-existing disorders.

2. Anesthetic: Depending on your desire and your doctor's suggestion, you will be given either local anesthetic or conscious sedation. Local anesthetic numbs the region, while conscious sedation allows you to rest throughout the treatment.

3. Sterilization: Once you are at ease, your doctor will find the vas deferens, the tubes that transport sperm from the testicles to the urethra. They will next create a tiny incision or puncture in the scrotum to get access to the vas deferens.

4. Vasectomy: Your doctor will stop the sperm's passage during ejaculation by cutting, sealing, or obstructing the vas deferens. This step is critical for successful sterilization.

5. Closure: Once the vasectomy is completed, your doctor will seal the incision site with dissolvable stitches or surgical glue. This closure promotes healthy healing while lowering the risk of infection.

6. Recovery: After the surgery, you will spend some time in the recovery area, where medical personnel will check your health. It is typical to feel slight soreness or swelling in the scrotal region, which may be treated with over-the-counter pain relievers and cold packs.

7. Follow-Up: Your doctor will provide you with post-procedure instructions, such as how to care for the incision site and when to arrange a follow-up consultation. It is essential to follow these instructions to guarantee a smooth recovery and the success of the vasectomy.

Understanding each phase of the vasectomy surgery will boost your confidence and prepare you for the treatment. If you have any questions or concerns, please address them with your healthcare practitioner.

Anesthesia Options And Pain Management

Choosing the appropriate anesthetic for your vasectomy may have a big influence on your comfort and overall experience. Here are the different alternatives and how they may help you manage discomfort.

1. **Local Anesthesia:** This technique entails injecting numbing medicine directly into the scrotal region, where the vasectomy will be performed. Local anesthetic prevents pain signals from reaching your brain, ensuring that you do not experience any discomfort throughout the operation. While you may experience pressure or pulling sensations, the treatment should be painless.

2. **Conscious Sedation:** For those who want to relax more throughout the process, conscious sedation may be prescribed. This entails delivering medicine via an IV line to generate a condition of tranquility and sedation. While you will stay cognizant and responsive, you will feel more calm and less aware that the procedure is going place.

3. **General Anesthesia:** In rare circumstances or for certain medical reasons, your doctor may suggest general anesthesia, which requires being entirely asleep during the treatment. This approach is usually

reserved for complicated patients or those who have trouble tolerating other types of anesthetic.

Regardless of the anesthetic option you choose, your healthcare practitioner will assure your safety and comfort during the vasectomy procedure. To make an educated choice, you must first discuss your preferences and any concerns you may have with your doctor.

Possible Dangers And Issues

While vasectomy is a safe and efficient method of permanent contraception, it, like any surgical operation, has risks and problems. Being aware of these dangers will allow you to make an educated choice and prepare for any issues. Here are some possible hazards related to vasectomy.

1. Bleeding: Although rare, significant bleeding may occur during or after vasectomy surgery. Your doctor will take steps to reduce this risk, such as applying pressure to the incision site and using safe surgical methods.

2. Infection at the incision site is another possible consequence of vasectomy. To limit this risk, keep the region clean and dry, adhere to post-procedure care instructions, and look for indications of infection, such as redness, swelling, or discharge.

3. **Chronic Pain:** Some people may endure chronic pain or discomfort in the scrotal region after a vasectomy, which is known as post-vasectomy pain syndrome (PVP). While uncommon, this ailment may have a major effect on quality of life and may need further medical examination and treatment.

4. **Sperm Granuloma:** A tiny lump known as a sperm granuloma might form at the place where the vas deferens are severed or sealed. While sperm granulomas are mostly innocuous, they may cause pain or inflammation and may need medical care if symptomatic.

5. Sperm Regrowth: In rare situations, the vas deferens may rejoin or grow back together after a vasectomy, resulting in the restoration of fertility. This condition, known as recanalization, might result in an unwanted pregnancy and may need further contraception methods.

Before having a vasectomy, you should talk to your doctor about the possible risks and problems. While the possibility of difficulties is minimal, being knowledgeable and prepared may help assure a positive result.

Post-Procedure Care Instructions

Following vasectomy surgery, effective post-procedure care is required to enhance healing, decrease pain, and limit the chance of problems. Here are some post-procedure guidelines to follow:

1. Rest and Recovery: Plan to relax for the first several days following vasectomy surgery, avoiding vigorous activity, heavy lifting, and excessive movement. Resting enables your body to recuperate and lowers the possibility of problems.

2. Ice Packs: Applying ice packs to the scrotum might help minimize swelling and pain after the surgery. Wrap the ice pack in a cloth or towel to avoid direct contact with the skin, then apply it for 15-20 minutes at a time, multiple times each day as required.

3. Pain Relief: Over-the-counter pain medicines such as acetaminophen (Tylenol) or ibuprofen (Advil, Motrin) might help lessen any discomfort or soreness after a vasectomy. Follow the specified dose and avoid aspirin, which might raise the risk of bleeding.

4. Wearing supportive underwear, such as briefs or snug-fitting boxer briefs, may assist offer extra comfort and support to the scrotal region while it heals. Avoid wearing tight or restricted clothes that may aggravate the incision site.

5. Keep the incision site clean and dry to avoid infection. Your doctor may give you specific instructions on how to care for the incision, such as gently cleaning it with soap and water and applying antibiotic ointment or dressing as needed.

6. **Follow-up visit:** Schedule a follow-up visit with your doctor as directed to ensure appropriate healing and to address any concerns or issues. Your doctor may undertake a post-procedure examination to ensure the vasectomy was successful.

Following these post-procedure care guidelines and communicating with your healthcare physician will help guarantee a smooth recovery and the success of the vasectomy. If you notice any unexpected symptoms or consequences, do not hesitate to see your doctor for advice and assistance.

CHAPTER 6

Recovery And Aftercare

Immediate Postoperative Care

To guarantee a successful recovery after a vasectomy, you must take excellent care of yourself right after. Your healthcare practitioner will offer particular advice based on your circumstances, but here are some broad suggestions. To begin, it is common to have soreness, edema, and bruising in the scrotal region after the treatment. To minimize swelling and relieve pain or discomfort, your doctor may prescribe using an ice pack wrapped in a towel. It is critical to follow your doctor's directions for pain management medicines. They may prescribe pain medicines or suggest over-the-counter remedies to alleviate any discomfort.

In addition, you should avoid intense activities, heavy lifting, and sexual activity for as long as your healthcare practitioner recommends. It is important to allow your body time to recover correctly, therefore adhere to any limits or suggestions advised. To limit the risk of infection, keep the incision site clean and dry. Your doctor may give you particular advice on how to care for the wound, such as covering it with gauze or applying antibiotic ointment.

Overcoming Pain And Uncomfort

Managing discomfort and suffering is an important part of the rehabilitation process after a vasectomy. While some soreness and swelling are expected following the treatment, there are some actions you may take to assist relieve pain and improve recovery. As previously stated, using an ice pack wrapped in a towel may help decrease swelling and relieve discomfort in the scrotal region. To assist manage any discomfort, your healthcare professional may prescribe using over-the-counter pain medicines such as ibuprofen or acetaminophen.

It is critical to follow your doctor's directions for pain management medication and avoid taking any drugs that may interfere with your existing prescriptions or medical problems. If you are experiencing severe or chronic pain, swelling, or other symptoms, contact your healthcare professional for more assistance. They may make additional suggestions or changes to your treatment plan as necessary to promote your comfort and well-being throughout the healing process.

Resuming Normal Activity

When it comes to returning to regular activities following a vasectomy, it's important to listen to your body and follow your doctor's instructions. While you may be anxious to resume your normal routine, it is important to allow your body the time it needs to recover correctly.

Your doctor will give you precise instructions for when you may safely resume activities like employment, exercise, and sexual activity.

In general, most men may resume work and mild activities within a few days to a week following the treatment, depending on the kind of job and how they feel. However, you should avoid heavy lifting, intense exercise, and sexual activity for as long as your healthcare practitioner recommends. Make sure to talk honestly with your doctor about any worries or questions you may have about returning to regular activities, and follow their advice to ensure a smooth recovery.

Long-Term Concerns For Sexual Health

After having a vasectomy, it is important to evaluate the long-term consequences for your sexual health. While a vasectomy is an extremely efficient method of permanent birth control, it is important to note that it does not protect against sexually transmitted diseases (STIs). If you are sexually active and at risk for STIs, you should continue to practice safe sex using condoms.

It's also crucial to be upfront with your spouse about your choice to get a vasectomy, as well as any worries or questions they may have. Some men may have changes in sexual function or desire after a vasectomy, although these are usually infrequent and transitory. If you have any concerns about your sexual health or notice any changes in your sexual function or libido, consult with your healthcare professional.

Additionally, it is important to have frequent check-ups with your healthcare practitioner to assess your general health and well-being. Your doctor may urge that you have regular follow-up consultations to check that your vasectomy was effective and to address any questions or concerns you may have regarding your sexual health. Staying knowledgeable and proactive about your sexual health can provide you with the peace of mind that comes with effective birth control and a healthy, enjoyable sex life.

CHAPTER 7

Possible Dangers And Issues

Common Risks Associated With Vasectomy

When choosing a medical treatment, it is important to understand the risks associated. While vasectomy is a typically safe and effective method of permanent contraception, it, like any surgical surgery, has hazards. One of the most prevalent concerns connected with vasectomy is groin discomfort or soreness after the surgery. This soreness usually goes away after a few days and may be treated with over-the-counter pain medications and icing the region.

Another typical complication is bruising and swelling around the scrotum. This is a common reaction to surgery and normally disappears on its own within a week or two.

Excessive bruising or swelling may suggest a more severe condition in rare situations, so keep a careful eye on these signs and call your doctor if you have any concerns.

Infection is another possible complication of vasectomy, albeit it is uncommon. To reduce the risk of infection, keep the surgical site clean and dry after the surgery. To lower the chance of infection even more, your doctor may prescribe antibiotics. If you have a fever, intense discomfort, significant swelling, or discharge from the surgery site, you should call your healthcare practitioner right once, as these might be signals of infection.

Rare Complications And How To Treat Them

While uncommon, there are a few possible problems connected with vasectomy that need medical intervention. A sperm granuloma is an uncommon condition that develops when sperm escapes from the vas deferens into the surrounding tissue, producing inflammation and discomfort. Sperm granulomas usually cure on their own, but if you have chronic discomfort or swelling, your doctor may prescribe anti-inflammatory drugs or, in rare situations, surgery.

A hematoma is an uncommon but deadly condition in which blood collects outside of a blood vessel. Hematomas may cause severe discomfort and swelling, requiring drainage or surgical intervention to treat. If you have extreme pain, swelling, or bruising in the scrotal region after vasectomy, call your healthcare professional right away, since these might be indicators of a hematoma.

Signs Of Postoperative Complications

Following a vasectomy, it is critical to constantly monitor your recovery and be alert for any indicators of post-operative problems. Some frequent symptoms of problems are:

1. Chronic or intensifying discomfort in the groin or scrotal area

2. Excessive swelling, bruising, or redness around the operative site

3. Fever or chills?

4. Difficulty Urinating or Blood in Urine

5. Infection signs include pus or drainage from the surgical site.

If you encounter any of these symptoms, you should contact your healthcare professional immediately. While most post-operative consequences are mild and readily addressed, others may need medical attention to prevent more severe problems from arising.

When To Seek Medical Attention?

In general, if you have any severe or persistent symptoms after a vasectomy, you should seek medical assistance right once.

This includes symptoms including acute pain, significant swelling or bruising, fever, and infection. In addition, if you have any questions about your recovery or notice any odd symptoms, please contact your healthcare practitioner for advice and assistance. If you have any reservations or worries regarding your post-operative recovery, it is always a good idea to seek medical assistance. Your healthcare professional is available to guide you through the healing process and ensure that you recuperate correctly after your vasectomy.

CHAPTER 8

Vasectomy Reversal

Overview Of The Vasectomy Reversal Procedure

Vasectomy reversal is a surgical technique designed to restore fertility in men who have previously had a vasectomy. The technique entails reconnecting the vas deferens, which transports sperm from the testicles to the urethra. It is normally done under local or general anesthesia in an outpatient environment, so you may usually go home the same day.

During the surgery, the physician makes tiny incisions in the scrotum to reach the vas deferens. Then they carefully find and reattach the severed or blocked ends of the vas deferens from the initial vasectomy. This delicate procedure requires painstaking accuracy, typically using microsurgical procedures to provide the best possible result.

After reconnecting the vas deferens, the surgeon will seal the incisions with dissolvable stitches. Recovery times vary, but most men may return to regular activities within a few days to a week after the treatment. However, it is critical to avoid heavy lifting or vigorous activity for a few weeks to allow for adequate recovery.

Success Rates And Factors Impacting Outcomes

Success rates for vasectomy reversal may vary based on several variables, including the surgeon's ability, the time since the initial vasectomy, and the existence of scar tissue or other issues. Men who have reversal sooner after their vasectomy have a greater success rate, ranging from 40% to more than 90%.

The kind of vasectomy done (e.g., basic or complicated), the length of the vas deferens remaining after the initial vasectomy, and the man's age and general health may all have an impact on the procedure's effectiveness.

Individuals contemplating vasectomy reversal should have reasonable expectations regarding the result. While the operation may successfully restore fertility in many men, there is no certainty of conception after reversal. Furthermore, even if sperm is available in the ejaculate during reversal, fertility may take many months to completely recover.

Alternatives For Vasectomy Reversal

Couples who are unable to conceive naturally after a vasectomy or vasectomy reversal have other choices for achieving conception. One frequent option is in vitro fertilization (IVF), which uses sperm extracted from the testicles to fertilize eggs in a laboratory environment.

This may be a helpful alternative for couples with male infertility or other difficulties conceiving naturally.

Another option is sperm retrieval coupled with intrauterine insemination (IUI), which involves injecting sperm from the testicles straight into the woman's uterus to aid in conception. This may be a less intrusive alternative than IVF and may be appropriate for certain couples based on their circumstances.

Emotional And Psychological Implications Of Reversal

Undergoing a vasectomy reversal may elicit a variety of feelings from both parties. Men may have emotions of excitement and anticipation about the chance of restoring fertility, as well as fear or ambiguity regarding the procedure's result. Men must communicate openly and honestly with their spouses about their sentiments and expectations about vasectomy reversal.

For couples who have been dealing with infertility, deciding to undergo vasectomy reversal may provide a newfound feeling of hope and possibilities. However, it is critical to be prepared for the emotional ups and downs that may occur throughout the process, including the chance of sadness if the surgery is not successful.

Counseling and support from healthcare practitioners, as well as other couples who have been through similar situations, may be very beneficial in navigating the emotional and psychological components of vasectomy reversal. Couples must rely on one another for support while being patient and resilient throughout the process, regardless of the result.

CHAPTER 9

Vasectomy Myths Busted

Addressing Common Misconceptions About Vasectomy

Misconceptions about vasectomy abound. Let's look at some of the most common misconceptions and discover the reality behind them.

Myth 1: A vasectomy causes erectile dysfunction

One of the most common myths is that vasectomy causes erectile dysfunction (ED). However, there is no scientific evidence to back this assertion. Vasectomy merely restricts the sperm-carrying tubes (vas deferens), not the blood vessels or nerves that cause erections. Men who have had a vasectomy are usually able to get and maintain erections.

Myth 2: Vasectomy reduces sexual pleasure

Another misconception claims that vasectomy reduces sexual pleasure. The truth is just the opposite. Men's sexual desire, performance, or feelings usually remain unchanged after a vasectomy. Some couples report an increase in sexual pleasure as a result of the lack of worry about unplanned pregnancies, resulting in a more comfortable and happy personal encounter.

Myth 3: Vasectomy is irreversible

While vasectomy is considered a permanent method of contraception, it is not completely irreversible. Men who want to restore fertility after a vasectomy might use techniques such as vasectomy reversal or sperm retrieval combined with in vitro fertilization (IVF). However, these methods do not guarantee success, and the likelihood of fertility restoration decreases with time. Consider vasectomy as a long-term choice and explore any reversibility issues with a healthcare physician before proceeding.

Myth 4: Vasectomy increases the risk of prostate cancer

There is a prevalent misperception that a vasectomy increases the risk of prostate cancer. However, multiple studies have not shown a conclusive association between vasectomy and prostate cancer. The American Urological Association and other prominent medical organizations have found that there is no solid evidence to support this assertion. Men seeking a vasectomy should be reassured that the procedure does not raise their risk of prostate cancer.

Distinguishing Fact From Fiction

Making educated judgments on vasectomy requires separating reality from myth. By dispelling these beliefs, people may eliminate unneeded worries and make informed decisions. To clear up any misunderstandings about vasectomy, talk with healthcare specialists, ask questions, and look for credible materials.

Clarifying Doubts And Concerns

Given the widespread misunderstandings regarding vasectomy, it is understandable for people to have reservations and worries. However, obtaining clarification from healthcare practitioners might assist in alleviating these doubts and make the decision-making process easier. Open discussion, a complete explanation of the treatment, and reasonable expectations are essential for overcoming uncertainties and reaping the advantages of vasectomy.

Promoting Informed Decision-Making

When contemplating a vasectomy, it is critical to empower educated decision-making. Individuals may make confident decisions that are in line with their reproductive objectives and lifestyle preferences by dispelling misconceptions, clearing concerns, and offering correct information.

CHAPTER 10

Life Following Vasectomy

Adjusting To Life After Vasectomy

Following a vasectomy, it is usual to experience a range of emotional and physical changes as you adjust to this new stage of your life. While the process itself is quite simple, it is critical to understand what to anticipate throughout the recovery time and beyond.

You may suffer scrotal pain, edema, and bruising immediately after the treatment. This is quite common and usually resolves within a few days to a week. Your doctor will give you advice on how to manage any discomfort, which may include taking over-the-counter pain medicines and using cold packs for the affected region.

Emotionally, some men may feel relieved that they no longer have to worry about unwanted pregnancies.

Others may feel hesitant or even sad, especially if they did not thoroughly evaluate the decision's long-term implications beforehand. Allow yourself time to absorb your feelings and, if necessary, address them freely with your spouse or a trusted healthcare practitioner.

As you return to regular activities, you may notice changes in your sexual function. While vasectomy does not affect desire or the capacity to achieve an erection, some men may notice a modest reduction in ejaculatory volume. This is because semen is mostly made up of fluid from the seminal vesicles and prostate, which are unaffected by the vasectomy. However, the overall sense of orgasm should be unchanged.

It is important to discuss freely with your spouse about any concerns or changes in your sexual health. Remember that vasectomy is a permanent method of contraception, so you must be confident in your choice and support each other throughout the transition time.

Effect On Sexual Health And Intimacy

One of the most prevalent worries among men contemplating a vasectomy is how it would impact their sexual health and intimacy. Fortunately, for the great majority of men, vasectomy does not affect sexual function or satisfaction.

Physiologically, a vasectomy simply disrupts sperm flow from the testes to the ejaculatory ducts. It does not affect testosterone production or the functioning of other sexual arousal and ejaculatory organs. As a consequence, most men have erections, orgasms, and the capacity to ejaculate properly after the operation.

Many couples report that having a vasectomy enhances their sexual connection since they are no longer concerned about the potential of unwanted pregnancy.

Couples who do not need to use other types of contraception, such as condoms or hormonal birth control, may feel more comfortable and spontaneous in their intercourse.

It's important to remember that everyone is unique, and some men may suffer temporary changes in sexual function or desire following a vasectomy. However, they are usually minor issues that resolve themselves with time.

If you have any worries about how a vasectomy may affect your sexual health or intimacy, please address them with your doctor. They may provide individualized advice and answer any questions or concerns you may have.

Family Planning Considerations

While vasectomy is an effective type of permanent contraception, you should carefully examine your family planning objectives before getting the operation.

For couples who are convinced they do not want to have any (or more) children, a vasectomy may give a piece of mind while eliminating the need for continued contraception. However, it is critical to have open and honest talks with your spouse about this choice, since it is usually irreversible.

If there is any ambiguity regarding future reproductive wishes, it may be worthwhile to consider alternate choices, such as long-acting reversible contraceptives (LARCs) for women and sperm banking for males. These options are more flexible and reversible than vasectomy.

Furthermore, it is essential to consider the emotional and psychological consequences of vasectomy for both yourself and your spouse. Some couples may find comfort in knowing that they have taken proactive steps to avoid unwanted pregnancies, but others may experience emotions of finality or loss.

Finally, the choice to have a vasectomy should be taken cautiously and collectively, taking into account the possible consequences for your relationship and future family planning. By openly and honestly discussing your choices, you may make an educated decision that is best for you and your partner.

Conclusion

To summarize, comprehending vasectomy requires a thorough awareness of the process, ramifications, and issues. This surgery, albeit easy to implement, has substantial implications for a man's reproductive destiny.

To begin, vasectomy is an effective method of permanent contraception because it obstructs the vas deferens, which is responsible for sperm transport. Its simplicity and minimal risk make it an appealing choice for males looking for a long-term contraceptive strategy. However, it is critical to understand that, although vasectomy is reversible in certain situations, the success of reversal treatments is not guaranteed, and anyone contemplating this option should carefully examine the risks and possible consequences.

Furthermore, the choice to get a vasectomy often incorporates psychological, social, and emotional factors. Men may have anxieties about their manhood, fertility, and sexual performance after surgery. Open communication with healthcare professionals, partners, and support networks is critical for addressing these issues and making informed choices.

Furthermore, the sociocultural environment around vasectomy warrants consideration. Cultural views, stigmas, and access to healthcare services all have the potential to impact people's contraceptive choices. Education and awareness efforts may help debunk misunderstandings, reduce stigma, and promote informed decisions about vasectomy and other contraceptive choices.

Furthermore, knowing the financial ramifications of a vasectomy is critical. While the initial cost of the treatment may seem high, it might be more cost-effective in the long term than alternative contraceptive options. Insurance coverage and access to subsidized healthcare services may influence cost and accessibility.

Finally, a thorough knowledge of vasectomy includes not just the medical components of the surgery, but also its psychological, social, and economic implications. Individuals may make informed choices about their reproductive health by participating in open discourse, seeking assistance, and taking into account all relevant aspects. Furthermore, healthcare practitioners play an important role in providing proper information, counseling, and support throughout the vasectomy procedure.

Finally, vasectomy is a personal decision that should be taken based on individual circumstances, choices, and values. Whether you choose permanent contraception or look into other options, educated decision-making and access to comprehensive reproductive healthcare services are critical.

THE END

www.ingramcontent.com/pod-product-compliance
Lightning Source LLC
Chambersburg PA
CBHW071841210526
45479CB00001B/232